Carlos Miguel Veiga
José Ferreira
Ana Portela

Cuttlefish Bone as a Biomaterial in Dentistry

Carlos Miguel Veiga
José Ferreira
Ana Portela

Cuttlefish Bone as a Biomaterial in Dentistry

A new material for alveolar preservation and bone regeneration

ScienciaScripts

Imprint
Any brand names and product names mentioned in this book are subject to trademark, brand or patent protection and are trademarks or registered trademarks of their respective holders. The use of brand names, product names, common names, trade names, product descriptions etc. even without a particular marking in this work is in no way to be construed to mean that such names may be regarded as unrestricted in respect of trademark and brand protection legislation and could thus be used by anyone.

Cover image: www.ingimage.com

This book is a translation from the original published under ISBN 978-613-9-63608-2.

Publisher:
Sciencia Scripts
is a trademark of
Dodo Books Indian Ocean Ltd. and OmniScriptum S.R.L publishing group

120 High Road, East Finchley, London, N2 9ED, United Kingdom
Str. Armeneasca 28/1, office 1, Chisinau MD-2012, Republic of Moldova, Europe
Printed at: see last page
ISBN: 978-620-7-67493-0

To my parents,

Thank you

I would like to thank my supervisor, Professor Ana Isabel Pereira Portela, for her availability and dedication. For her contribution, help, suggestions, ideas and continuous encouragement to carry out research, even in times of adversity.

To Professor José Maria da Fonte Ferreira for providing the samples used in this monograph, as well as for his knowledge, support and accompaniment throughout the work.

My special thanks go to Professor Manuel Augusto Gomes de Oliveira Azenha for making the equipment available at the Department of Chemistry and Biochemistry of the Faculty of Sciences of the University of Porto, as well as for his help in handling the technical means.

To Professor José António Ferreira Lobo Pereira for his help with the statistical treatment and interpretation of the results.

To my sister for her friendship and support, for accompanying me at every stage.

I would like to thank my parents. For being my compass, for supporting me in every aspect of my life, for always encouraging me to work towards my goals and providing me with all the means to do so.

General Index

Summary

Introduction: Cuttlefish bone is a biomaterial that has been studied for use in health areas such as orthopaedics and dentistry. Various in vitro and in vivo tests have been carried out, as well as other tests regarding the cytotoxicity and biological and mechanical characterisation of the material. However, given its origin and before moving on to tests on human patients, this material needs further study, particularly with regard to the detection and quantification of heavy metals present in its composition.

Objectives: The aim was to detect and quantify the heavy metals present in cuttlefish bone before and after hydrothermal processing, in order to certify its safety for implantation in the alveolar bone of patients after tooth extraction and for the purpose of filling bone defects.

Materials and methods: Cuttlefish bone samples were taken from specimens caught off the coast of Esmoriz in January and March 2016. The samples were taken from two different municipal markets. The samples were divided into four groups: Groups A1 and B1 (with material not subjected to hydrothermal treatment from Mercado de Santiago in group A1 and Mercado Municipal de Espinho in group B1) and Groups A2 and B2 (with material subjected to hydrothermal treatment from Mercado de Santiago in group A2 and Mercado Municipal de Espinho in group B2). The samples were reduced to powder, digested using a solution of concentrated nitric acid (65%) and subjected to detection and quantification of heavy metals using flame atomic absorption spectrometry (for zinc, copper, cadmium and lead) and cold vapour reduction atomic absorption spectrometry (for mercury).

Results: The average concentrations found in the samples were lower than the maximum values established by the European Commission (in relation to muscle intended for ingestion) and the maximum permitted concentrations established by the Food and Drug Administration for all the metals tested, except for lead and cadmium.

Conclusion: Zinc, mercury, lead, cadmium and copper were detected in all the samples tested. Although the average lead concentrations were higher than the maximum values set by the European

Commission and the Food and Drug Administration and the average cadmium concentrations were higher than the maximum values set by the Food and Drug Administration, this does not mean that the material is excluded from biomedical applications in dentistry and orthopaedics.

Future work could include co-cultures with osteoblasts and osteoclasts, quantifying the heavy metals present in the culture medium that may have been released by the hydroxyapatite obtained by hydrothermal processing of cuttlefish bone and methods of processing the material in order to reduce the concentrations of lead and cadmium if they are released from the sample into the physiological environment.

Keywords: cuttlebone, bone crest preservation, alveolar preservation, bone regeneration, biomaterials

CHAPTER 1

Introduction

Tooth extraction is one of the most frequently performed medical and dental procedures and the dimensional changes to the alveolar ridge that occur as a result of this clinical act are well documented in the literature. (1) It has already been shown that buccal horizontal bone loss can reach 56%, lingual bone loss can reach 30% (1, 2) and the total horizontal reduction of the alveolar ridge can reach 50%. (1, 3) Tan et al. (4) concluded that horizontal bone loss is greater than vertical bone loss. These changes are important when drawing up a treatment plan for prosthetic rehabilitation, taking into account the possible complications to be expected during rehabilitation. (4)

Today, implants are widely used and have become a regular part of most dentists' daily lives. The level of crestal bone surrounding the implant is of the utmost importance in determining its successful osseointegration, while preserving the height of marginal bone is extremely important for its long-term survival. Various approaches have been described in the literature to prevent bone loss. (5) Loss of bone crest height leads to greater bacterial accumulation, which results in secondary peri-implantitis, which can subsequently lead to a loss of bone support, causing excessive occlusal loads on the implant which, in turn, cause even greater bone crest loss. (5, 6) This vicious cycle will ultimately lead to implant failure.

Several studies (1, 4, 7, 11-16) have shown that there is less resorption of the alveolar ridge when preservation techniques are used compared to cases where no material is inserted into the alveolus immediately after extraction. There are various materials available on the market - but most of them, as well as being expensive, are used for regeneration itself and not for preserving the dental alveolus.

It is therefore important to find a material that not only preserves the alveolus as much as possible after extraction, but is also inexpensive enough for patients to accept its use immediately after a tooth extraction, and which the general dentist can use in most tooth extractions for subsequent rehabilitation of the edentulous space.

Cuttlefish bone, also known in the literature as cuttlebone or cuttlefish bone, is a lightweight, porous material that has received considerable attention in the literature over the last few decades. It belongs to a class of ultra-light biomaterials with high rigidity and cell permeability, which allows cuttlefish to maintain neutral buoyancy in environments of considerable depth. (17) It is inexpensive to obtain, is of biological origin and is available worldwide. (18) In addition to these advantages, cuttlefish bone is also compatible with other types of bone structures and has a high osteoinductive capacity. (19)

CHAPTER 2

This study aims to detect the presence of the heavy metals zinc, copper, cadmium, lead and mercury in samples of cuttlefish bone caught off the Portuguese coast.

Different samples were analysed in order to assess whether the effect of the hydrothermal processing to which the material is subjected and the place where the samples were taken alter the concentrations detected.

By detecting and quantifying these elements, the aim was to ascertain whether the heavy metal content could pose a risk when the material is implanted in the dental socket immediately after tooth extraction in human patients.

CHAPTER 3

Material and methods

The samples used in this study were obtained from fresh cuttlefish caught off the coast of Esmoriz (Table I). They were collected in January and March 2016 from two municipal markets in the Aveiro district. After extracting the bone, it was cleaned with running water and dried in the air.

Table I - Description of the samples taken

Date of receipt and origin of the sample	Sample	Untreated ($CaCO_3$)	Processed (Calcium Phosphates)
March 2016 Mercado Santiago, Aveiro	1.1	X	
	1.2	X	
	1.3	X	
	1.4	X	
	1.5	X	
	1.6	X	
	1.7		X
	1.8		X
	1.9		X
	1.10		X
January 2016 Espinho Municipal Market, Aveiro	2.1	X	
	2.2	X	
	2.3	X	
	2.4	X	
	2.5	X	
	2.6	X	
	2.7		X
	2.8		X
	2.9		X
	2.10		X
	2.11		X
	2.12		X

Reduction of bone to powder and HT processing

After drying, part of the collected bone was ground into powder using a pestle and mortar. The other part was hydrothermally processed using an autoclave. For this HT processing, several portions of cuttlefish bone were placed in an autoclave (made to order, in stainless steel with a Teflon inner chamber; the outer cover is fixed with 4 screws and the watertightness is maintained with a Viton O-ring). The HT transformation was carried out at a heating rate of 5°C/min up to 200°C, for 48 hours at this temperature. After two days, the autoclave was opened to remove the samples. The transformed samples were then sintered in an electric furnace (Termolab, Portugal), according to the following heat treatment: 2°C/min up to 500°C, 5°C/min between 500-1100°C, 1h plateau at this temperature, followed by natural cooling inside the furnace to a temperature close to room temperature. After HT processing, the samples were ground into powder using a pestle and mortar.

Both the HT processing and the reduction of the bone to powder were carried out in the laboratories of the Materials and Ceramics Engineering Department at the University of Aveiro.

The samples were therefore divided into four groups:

Group A1: HT unprocessed bone from Mercado de Santiago

Group A2: Bone with HT processing from Mercado de Santiago

Group B1: Unprocessed HT bone from Espinho Market

Group B2: Bone with HT processing from Mercado de Espinho

Sample digestion

The samples from each group were weighed using an analytical balance (Mettler Toledo, model AG245, Switzerland) (A1: 5.2834 ± 0.0001 g; A2: 4.4426 ± 0.0001 g; B1: 6.6696 ± 0.0001 g; B2: 4.4556 ± 0.0001 g). The samples were then transferred to Erlenmeyer flasks (Figure 1), where 65% concentrated nitric acid was added.

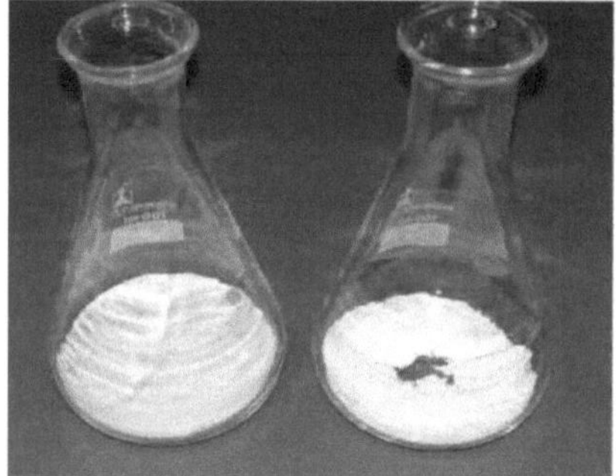

Figura 1 - Samples in *Erlenmeyer flasks* before adding concentrated nitric acid. On the left, unprocessed cuttlefish bone from group A1. On the right, cuttlefish bone with HT treatment from group A2.

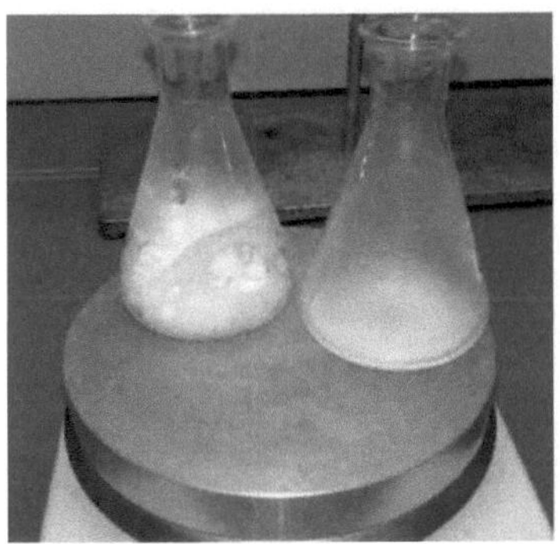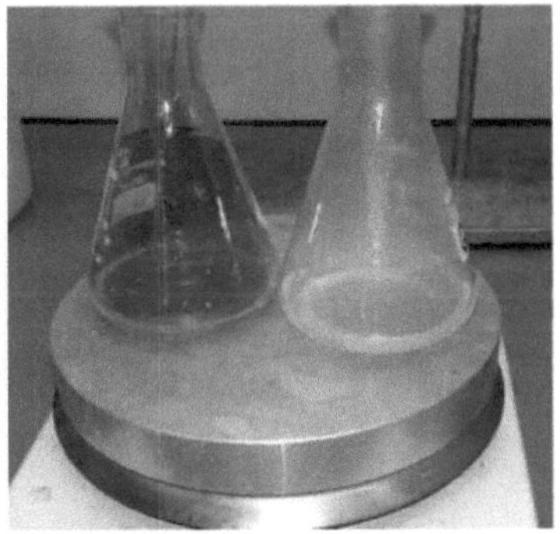

Figura 2   - Samples immediately after the addition of concentrated nitric acid (left) and after 1 hour of digestion (right)

The matrazes were placed on a hotplate where the solution was heated to boiling point (Figure 2). In the matzahs with the processed samples (groups A2 and B2), small particles of undigested material were observed even after 2 hours of digestion, which were considered impurities, filtered and discarded before analysis by spectrometry.After digestion, distilled water was added to each of the matzahs until 100 mL of solution was obtained.

Analysis by atomic absorption spectrometry with flame atomisation and mercury cold vapour reduction

After digesting the bone, the heavy metals present were detected and quantified by flame atomisation atomic absorption spectrometry for Zinc (Zn), Copper (Cu), Cadmium (Cd) and Lead (Pb) using a flame atomic absorption spectrometer (Perkin Elmer Instruments, model AAnalyst 200, USA) (Figure 3). Before analysing each of the metals, calibration was carried out using standard solutions of known concentration for each of the metals analysed. There were 6 readings for Pb, Cu and Cd and 3 readings for Zn, after which the average was calculated.

To detect and quantify Hg, the cold vapour mercury reduction atomic absorption spectrometry technique was used (Perkin Elmer Instruments, MHS-15, USA), with NaBH4 as the reducing agent and argon as the carrier gas. Three readings were taken and the average was calculated.

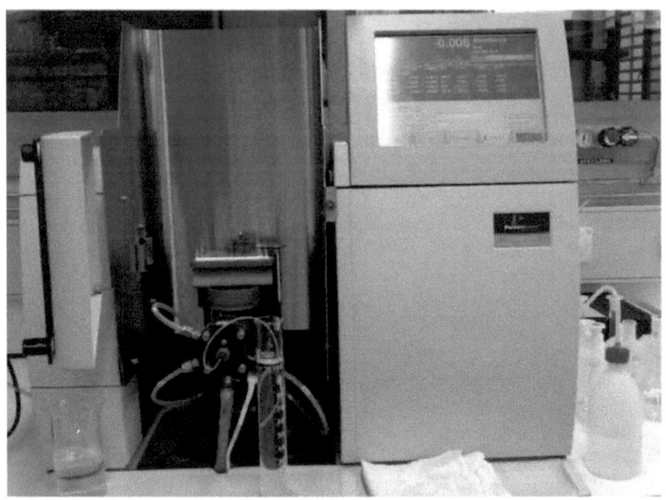

Figure 3 - Flame atomic absorption spectroscopy

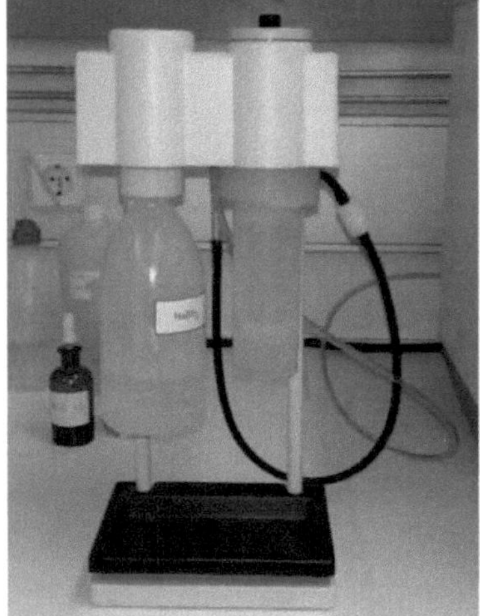

Figure 4 - Hg reduction system

Statistical analysis

The SPSS software programme for Windows 10 - IBM SPSS Statistics 23.0 (USA) and the Microsoft Office 2013 software programme (USA) were used for statistical processing. The Mann-Whitney non-parametric test ($p<0.05$) was applied to assess the differences in concentrations between processed and unprocessed samples and between samples taken at different locations.

CHAPTER 4

Results

Table II shows that all the samples analysed detected the presence of the elements investigated. However, the values varied between samples with and without treatment, as well as depending on where they were collected.

Table II - mean and standard deviation of heavy metal concentrations

Metal	A1	A2	B1	B2
Pb (µg/g)	33,17 (4,88)	18,17 (1,83)	27,83 (1,72)	17,83 (3,60)
Zn (µg/g)	19,33 (0,58)	22,67 (0,58)	33,67 (0,58)	43,33 (1,15)
Cu (µg/g)	4,83 (0,16)	5,18 (0,26)	4,00 (0,09)	4,17 (0,08)
Cd (µg/g)	<0.4 (N.D)	1,38 (0,30)	< 0.3 (N.D.)	0,75 (0,23)
Hg (µg/g)	< 28 (N.D.)	< 34 (N.D.)	< 22 (N.D)	< 34 (N.D.)

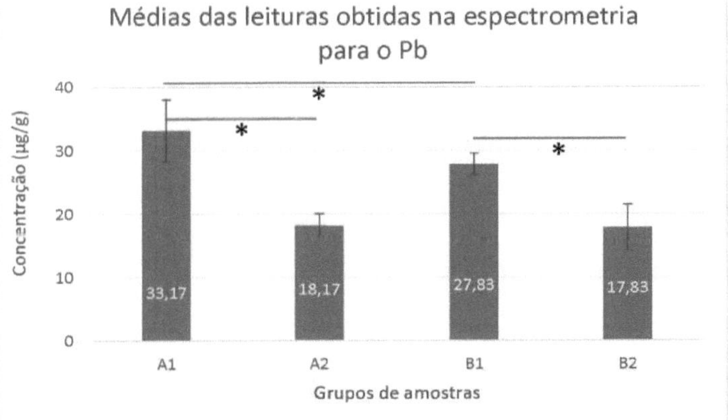

Graph 1 - Comparison of mean Pb concentrations. The asterisk indicates statistically significant differences between the groups ($p<0.05$).

The untreated samples had the highest Pb concentrations compared to the hydrothermally processed ones. Of the untreated samples, those collected at the Mercado de Santiago (A1) had the highest average concentration (Table II, Graph 1).

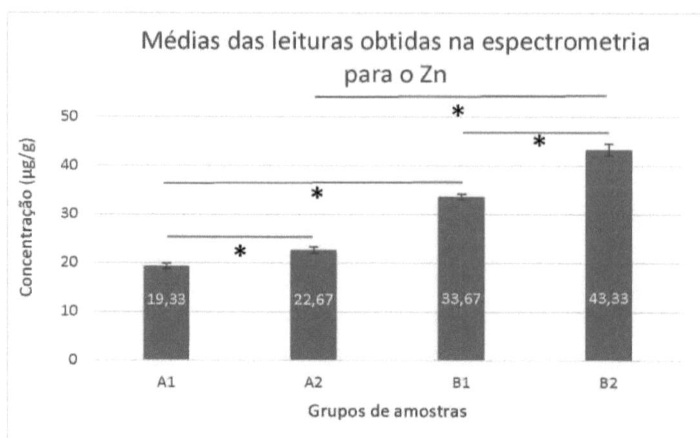

Graph 2 - Comparison of mean Zn concentrations. The asterisk indicates statistically significant differences between the groups (p<0.05).

The treated samples had higher average Zn concentrations than the unprocessed ones. The samples collected at the Espinho market that had been hydrothermally processed (B2) had a higher average concentration (Table II, Graph 2).

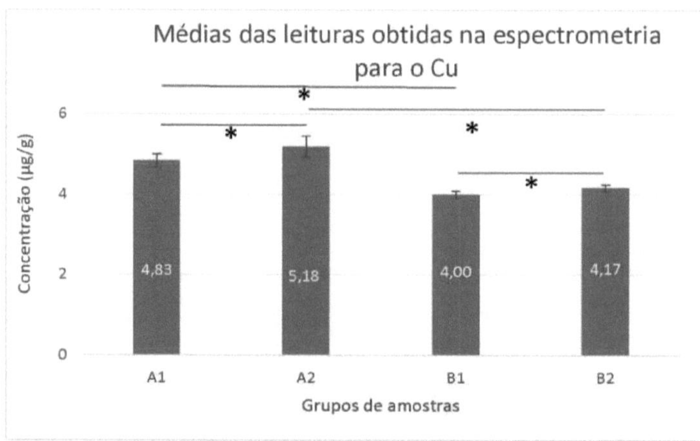

Graph 3 - Comparison of mean Cu concentrations. The asterisk indicates statistically significant differences between the groups (p<0.05).

The treated samples had higher average Cu concentrations than the unprocessed ones. The samples collected at the Mercado de Santiago that were hydrothermally processed (A2) were the ones with the highest average concentration (Table II, Graph 3).

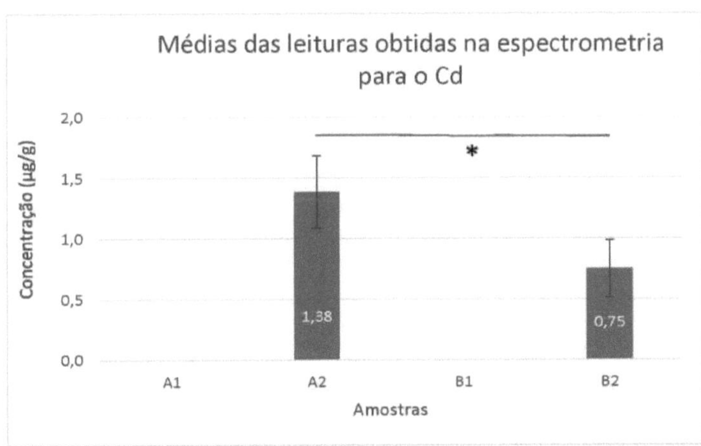

Graph 4 - Comparison of mean Cd concentrations. The asterisk indicates statistically significant differences between the groups (p<0.05).

The average Cd values of the samples in groups A1 and B1 are not shown in Graph 4, as the readings taken were below the detection limit for the sample masses used (concentrations of <0.4 µg/g were detected in group A1 and <0.3 µg/g in group B1). The average concentrations were higher in the groups of hydrothermally processed samples, with those obtained at the Mercado de Santiago (A2) recording a higher average (Table II, Graph 4).

With regard to Hg, in the readings taken, the values detected were below the detection limits for the sample masses used, in all the sample groups (concentrations <28 ng/g were detected in group A1, <34 ng/g in groups A2 and B2 and <22 ng/g in group B1) (Table II).

CHAPTER 5

Discussion

Cuttlefish bone as a biomaterial

Cuttlefish bone is made up of two parts: the outermost - the dorsal layer - is quite rigid and dense, made up of plates and columns of aragonite, protecting the innermost structure - the lamellar matrix - an extremely porous structure (with up to 90% porosity), with channels that allow intercommunication between the pores (Figure 5). (17, 18, 20, 21) According to Wiesmann et. al. (22), the pores of a bone graft must be between 200 and 500 ^m in diameter for revascularisation and bone restructuring to occur. Since the pore diameter of cuttlefish bone varies between 200 and 600 μm (Figures 6 and 7) (23), it is valid to hypothesise that this material could be a suitable graft for harbouring and maintaining tissue biological activities (24), such as bone tissue growth and vascularisation. (18) The lamellar matrix is essentially made up of aragonite (18), a crystallised form of calcium carbonate (17), surrounded by a layer of organic matter (17, 20, 21) made up essentially of a layer of β-chitin. (17) This porous structure enables physical contact between the host tissues and facilitates the exchange of minerals and vascularisation. (20)

In Bioengineering, scaffolds are defined as solid, porous biomaterials designed to fulfil various functions, including promoting interaction between cells and the biomaterial, cell adhesion, proliferation and differentiation, and biodegradation at a controlled rate, close to that of the tissue regeneration of interest (11).

Biominerals with complex structures such as cuttlebone (20) have been studied due to their potential applications as scaffolds in bone regeneration engineering. (25-27) Due to the chemical, physical and mechanical characteristics of this material, a wide range of new applications have been investigated. (17)

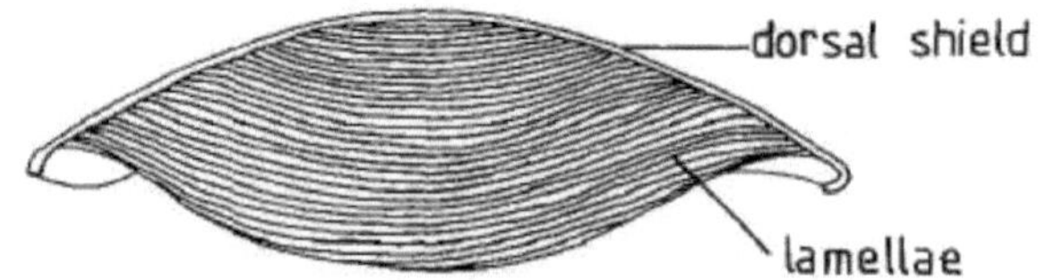

Figura 5 - representative diagram of a cross-section of the cuttlefish bone. Adapted from (20)

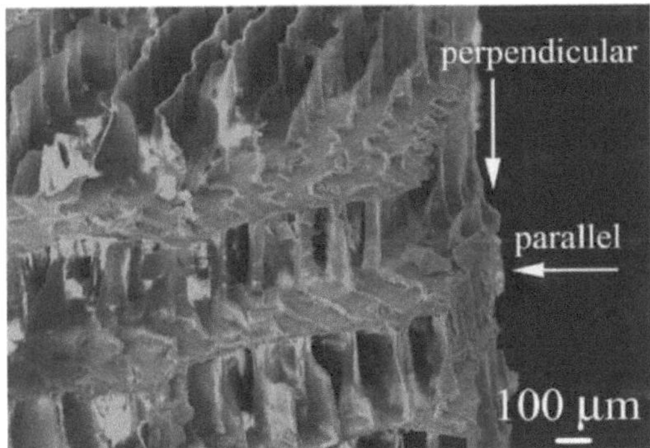

Figura 6 - Lamellar porous structure of cuttlefish bone. The arrows indicate parallel and perpendicular orientation. Adapted from (18)

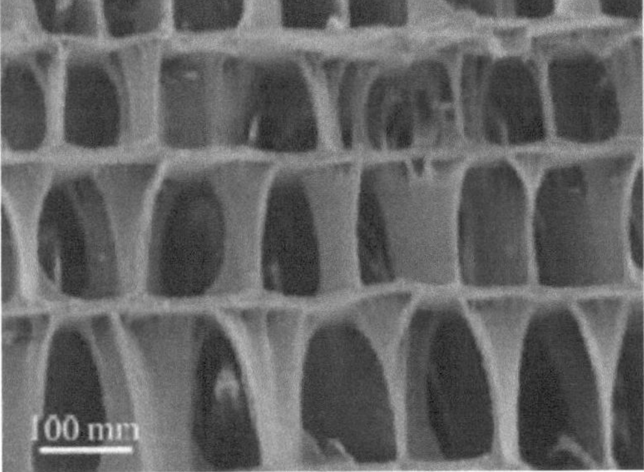

Figura 7 - Detail of the lamellar structure of cuttlefish bone. Adapted from (17)

In 2007, Yildirim et. al. (28) investigated the compatibility of unprocessed cuttlefish bone with human tissue. Together with their collaborators, they found that the mineral composition of cuttlefish bone is compatible with human tissues and suggested that this material as a scaffold for bone tissue regeneration was worthy of further study in the future. (17) In 2009 and 2010, Jasso-Gastinel et. al. al. (29) and Garcia-Enriquez et. al. (30) investigated the use of cuttlefish bone in acrylic bone cements and found good osseointegration without any evidence of secondary infection during their in vivo tests on rabbits. They found that the mechanical properties of bone cement with 30% cuttlefish bone in its composition were within the standard criteria applicable to this type of cement, and were comparable to commercial presentations of marketed bone cements. (17)

HT processing

Another approach to the use of cuttlefish bone in tissue engineering applications involves HT processing of the aragonite, converting it into hydroxyapatite (HA), a calcium phosphate ceramic that

17

has proven to be suitable for this type of use. (17) In 2005 and 2006, Rocha et. al. (18, 23) and in 2007 Kannan et. al. (31) used HT processing to produce tissue scaffolds. (17) This was the type of processing used in this work to transform the samples.

Below, the chemical equation that represents the transformation of cuttlebone aragonite ($CaCO3$) into HA ($Ca10(PO4)6(OH)2$) through HT processing. (31)

$$10CaCO_3 + 6(NH_4)_2HPO_4 + 2H_2O \rightarrow Ca_{10}(PO_4)_6(OH)_2 + 6(NH_4)_2CO_3 + 4H_2CO_3$$

Even after HT processing, the porous structure is preserved and the material's channel microstructure is not altered (Figure 8). (23)

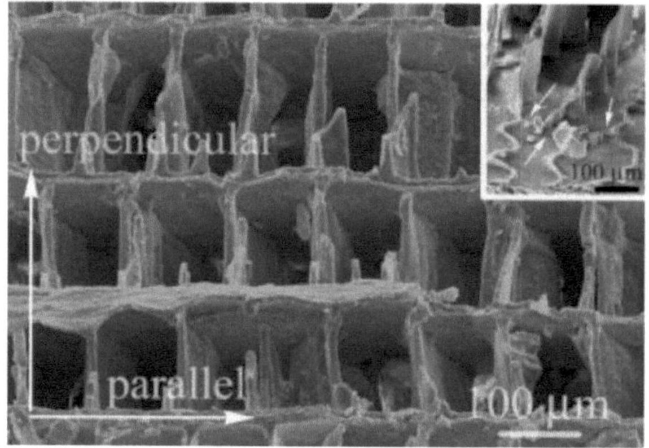

Figura 8 - Lamellar porous structure of cuttlefish bone. The dimensions of the channels **observed were ~ 80 µm in width and = 100 µm in height. This photograph** belongs to a sample after 24h of HT processing. Adapted from (23).

The transformation process produces mixed carbonated HA of type A and B, similar to the composition of human bone, in which just 1 hour of HT processing is enough to transform aragonite into HA (18,23).

A major advantage of this ceramic scaffold is that it can meet bioactivity requirements, as well as any modelling requirements which, if desired, can be tailor-made for each clinical case - especially in the case of badly damaged bones. (18)

The material can be machined to take on any desired shape (Figure 9), at any of its processing stages (before or after sintering), making it possible to meet the most demanding technical requirements in terms of speed, customisation and making a fragment to be implanted, which is particularly relevant, for example, in cases of broken bones due to road accidents (18) or in order to adapt to the shape of an alveolus after tooth extraction. Calcium phosphate blocks (such as HA obtained from the HT processing of cuttlefish bone) can fill bone defects with a predictable shape and size, but do not achieve good contact between the surface of the block and the bone - in this case, the use of the material in the form of granules is the most appropriate, adapting the size of the granules to the size of the most common defects (in dentistry, the granules should be < 1 mm in diameter) (7, 32).

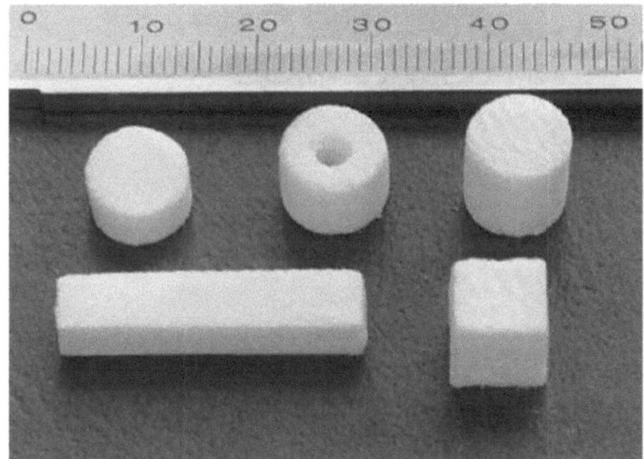

Figura 9 - *Scaffolds* can be machined to various shapes easily, quickly and at any stage of processing (scale in mm). Adapted from (18).

In addition to versatility in terms of shape, these scaffolds can have varying degrees of bioactivity and solubility - they can range from practically insoluble HA to soluble calcium phosphate (the ionic product of whitlockite), depending on the clinical case objectives. Materials with smaller grains or a higher glass phase content are more soluble than more crystalline materials with larger grains. To control the degree of solubility, it is only necessary to vary the sintering temperature. The sintering temperature significantly influences the microstructure of scaffolds (18).

The results of the in vitro tests carried out by Rocha et. al. (18) with osteoblasts show that the scaffolds produced from hydrothermally processed cuttlefish bone are suitable for biological applications. There was also rapid and pronounced HA formation on the surface of the scaffolds after immersion in SBF for 1 and 2 weeks (18). Optimum osteoblast proliferation and very good biocompatibility with osteoblasts were also recorded. (18) These data are in line with the conclusions of the experimental study by Okumuş et. *al. (26),* carried out in 2005 on New Zealand rabbits. As

19

well as being bioactive (33), the material is also osteoinductive (34).

Rocha et. al. (18) concluded that HA obtained from cuttlefish bone has an excellent biomineralisation capacity and, according to studies with materials incorporating HA (35, 36), the presence of HA increases the viability of osteoblasts and does not affect the production of alkaline phosphatase (AP). (18) However, according to Hongmin et. al. (34), AP activity is higher in hydrothermally processed cuttlefish bone than in unprocessed cuttlefish bone. Figure 10 shows the considerable increase in the viability/proliferation of osteoblasts in the presence of powders obtained by grinding scaffolds after HT processing for 24 hours (24 hour group) and HT processing for 24 hours followed by sintering at 1250°C (1250°C group). Group A (graph on the left) represents the analysis of cell viability using the MTT reduction assay and group B (graph on the right) represents the analysis of cell viability using FA production with NBT-BCIP analysis. (18)

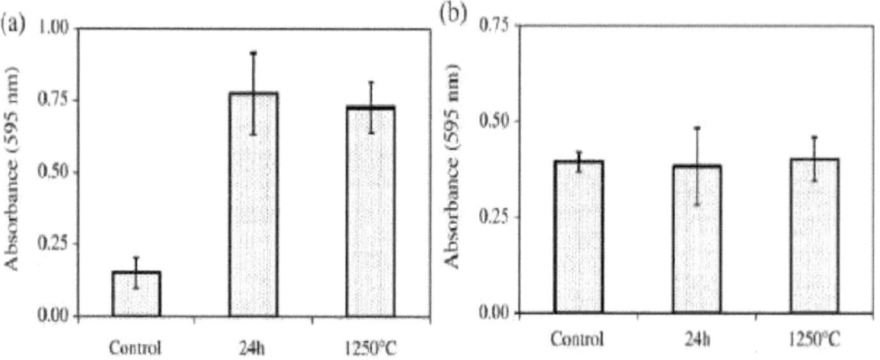

Figura 10 - Results of osteoblast viability/proliferation after 72h of incubation. Results represent duplicates of 8 (a) and 6 (b) different experiments (p < 0.05). Adapted from (18).

The study carried out by Hongmin et. al. (34) in 2015 found that, after 13 days, the mesenchymal stem cells in HA formed from cuttlefish bone increased the amount of osteocalcin and FA, compared to cuttlefish bone without any type of HT processing. (34) In vivo studies have shown that HA obtained from the HT treatment of cuttlefish bone was able to induce ectopic bone formation, which was not the case with unprocessed cuttlefish bone. (34) Compared to the control (unprocessed material), cuttlefish bone subjected to HT treatment (scaffold) increased the viability of osteoblasts and did not change the production of FA (Figure 11). (23) HT processing could therefore be advantageous in terms of the material's clinical performance compared to unprocessed cuttlefish bone, such as that used in **2005 by Okumu§** et. *al. (26)* in their experiment with New Zealand rabbits.

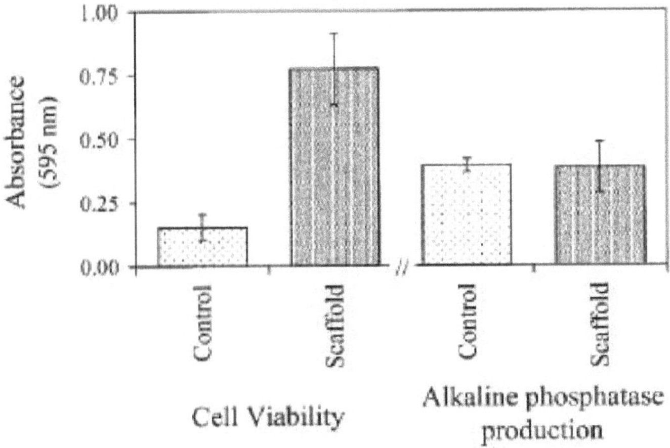

Figura 11   - Osteoblasts were placed in contact with the *scaffolds and* subjected to 24 hours of HT. After 24 hours of incubation, cell viability/proliferation was assessed by MTT analysis and FA production by NBT-BCIP analysis. The results represent average values. Adapted from (23).

According to the study by **Orkumuç et.** *al. (26) the* data obtained from radiographic examination, histological analysis, magnetic resonance imaging and scintigraphy revealed that cuttlefish bone without HT processing ranked second in terms of best performance in the bone healing process among the 4 materials tested (demineralised bone matrix, cuttlebone without HT processing, cancellous bovine bone and calcium triphosphate), revealing that this material has osteoconductive capacity, is resorbable (as it does not undergo HT processing, aragonite is not converted into HA) and does not interfere with the graft integration process. Furthermore, the absence of giant cells in response to the exposure of host tissues to this material shows that cuttlefish bone may well be considered a new option for use as a xenograft (26).

Nine years after the **study by Okumu§ et.** *al.* (26), Dogan **et.** *al.* (24) carried out a similar trial, but with a significantly larger sample and the introduction of a control group. The authors of this study, based on the data from the clinical and histological analyses, concluded that cuttlefish bone appears to be a compatible material that manages to establish bone union earlier without causing excessive oxidative damage. Due to the high degree of vascularisation seen in the cuttlefish bone group and the acceleration of osteogenesis and osseointegration, cuttlefish bone was considered the best material in this study. (24)

Heavy metals

Heavy metals are all those that have a density of more than 5 g/cm^3 and cause adverse effects on the environment and living beings. (37) Over the last few decades, several human actions have introduced significant quantities of polluting metals, both stable and radioactive, into marine environments. Many of these contaminants are removed from seawater through physical, chemical and biological processes, the latter including incorporation into marine organisms. (38, 39)

Despite the cuttlefish's short life cycle, its strong ability to accumulate a wide variety of metals in its tissues has already been demonstrated (40-43).

HA is known to have a tendency to accumulate various metals and metalloids by adsorption, due to the characteristics of its surface. This adsorption mechanism is based on ion exchange, involving Ca ions^{2+}, PO_4^{3-} and H$^+$ from HA. (44, 45) Several studies have shown an excellent capacity for retaining and stabilising Cd, Zn, Cu and Pb in the structure of HA (45-71), revealing the binding affinity of these metals to HA.

Therefore, given the biological origin of the HA produced from cuttlefish bone, whose marine habitat contains heavy metals, doubts have been raised about the amount of these metals that may be present in the reaction product, as well as the risk that these metals may entail when implanting the material in human bone and its possible migration into the biological environment.

While the mineral portion of natural bone can be remodelled by osteoclast action, sintered HA is not biodegradable and is not resorbed by osteoclasts. (32, 72-75) Studies indicate that the dissolution rate of sintered HA is low (76-78), preserving the outline of sintered HA granules even 4 weeks after being implanted in animal models. (75) However, one of the properties of HA obtained by HT treatment of cuttlefish bone is that it is possible to obtain various degrees of solubility by varying the sintering temperature. (18)

Given the non-existent resorption of sintered HA by osteoclasts and the strong bond that these divalent metals have with HA, it is hypothesised that the release of these heavy metals into the body is nil or very residual, remaining in the structure of the HA scaffold. The speciation of these metals is crucial when assessing their mobility and potential toxicity, as their behaviour is highly dependent on their chemical form and binding states. (79-82) In in vivo studies in which cuttlefish bone was implanted in bone defects (24, 26), no adverse effects related to local or systemic heavy metal toxicity were observed. However, there is a need for a longer, more targeted analysis of the toxicity caused by these elements.

In a study carried out on animal models (83), the effect of Cu and Zn on cell viability was analysed, and it was concluded that at the concentrations used in the tests, there were no significant differences compared to the control group; in fact, in the case of Zn, a significantly statistical increase in cell viability was observed. Thus, the presence of heavy metals in certain concentrations may not only have harmful effects, but may even be beneficial for bone metabolism, so their presence in materials for bone regeneration should be carefully considered.

Zn recorded average concentrations below the WHO daily reference values. (92)

The average concentrations of Cu and Hg in the samples analysed were lower than the limits set by the EC (9, 10) in cuttlefish muscle intended for ingestion, lower than the daily exposure value allowed by the FDA and lower than the maximum daily values allowed for the element when integrating drugs and derivatives as an impurity, valid for parenteral administration. (8)

The average Pb concentrations were higher than those permitted by the EC (9, 10) in cuttlefish muscle intended for ingestion and higher than the daily exposure value permitted by the FDA and higher than the maximum daily values permitted for the element when integrating drugs and derivatives as an impurity, valid for administration by parenteral route. (8)

With regard to Cd, the average concentrations in the samples tested were lower than the limits set by the EC (9, 10) in cuttlefish muscle intended for ingestion, lower than the daily exposure value allowed by the FDA but higher than the maximum daily values allowed for the element when integrating drugs and derivatives as an impurity, valid for administration by parenteral route. (8)

Although Pb and Cd show average concentrations higher than those permitted, it should be borne in mind that the reference values used refer to the parenteral administration route when the material is actually implanted, assuming 100 per cent bioavailability, which is not the case in vivo. In addition, the high affinity of metals for HA should be taken into account, as well as the low degree of resorption of the **scaffold** and, therefore, the residual release of metals into the biological environment.

HT processing and concentrations of heavy metals analysed

Between groups A1 and A2 and between groups B1 and B2 there were statistically significant differences (p<0.05) in the concentrations of the metals Pb, Cu and Zn, with an increase in the concentration of Cu and Zn in the processed samples and a decrease in the concentration of Pb. Thus, HT treatment seems to significantly affect the concentration of metals in the samples, with the decrease in the concentration of Pb standing out as a clear advantage of HT processing.

This variation can be explained by the tendency of the metals present in the initial material to adsorb to the surface of the calcium phosphate phases formed during HT processing or possibly to enter their structure and remain in the processed material, thus increasing their concentration. The presence of organic matter in the composition of the initial material, which disappears when it is processed, also helps to explain the differences observed.

Collection site and concentrations of heavy metals analysed

Between the groups of unprocessed samples taken at different locations (A1 and B1) there were statistically significant differences **(p<0.05) in the** concentrations of Pb, Cu and Zn, with group A1 recording higher average concentrations of Pb and Cu and lower concentrations of Zn.

Between the groups of processed samples taken at different locations (A2 and B2) there were statistically significant differences (p<0.05) in the concentrations of Cu, Cd and Zn, with group A2 recording higher average concentrations of Cu and Cd, but a lower average concentration of Zn. The differences in the average concentration of Pb were not statistically significant **(p>0.05)** between groups A2 and B2.

Bearing these values in mind, it will be important to specify where the material is collected in order to reduce the variability in the composition of the biomaterial to be implanted.

CHAPTER 6

Conclusions

The assessment of the heavy metals present in the cuttlefish bone samples used in this study revealed some variability in the parameters analysed:

- The different metals are found in different concentrations, with Pb showing values above those recommended by regulatory institutions; Cd is within the values recommended by two of the regulatory institutions and higher only with regard to parenteral administration. Cu and Hg showed values within the range permitted by these institutions;

- The hydrothermal treatment of the samples is favourable with regard to all the values analysed, especially the reduction in Pb values.

- The location where the samples were taken influences the values for the different heavy metals quantified.

The literature states that the pharmacokinetics, bioavailability and absorption rate of metals, as well as the degree of solubility of the scaffold are extremely important data when assessing the danger of the metals included in the material to be implanted, and with the aim of confirming and trying to solve the problem raised by the results obtained in this study, we suggest that future work should be carried out on co-cultures with osteoblasts and osteoclasts, quantifying the heavy metals present in the culture medium that may have been released by the HA obtained by HT processing of cuttlefish bone.

The use of additional material processing methods to reduce lead and cadmium concentrations is recommended if they are released from the scaffold into the physiological environment.

Bibliographical references

1.   Horowitz R, Holtzclaw D, Rosen PS. A Review on Alveolar Ridge Preservation Following Tooth Extraction. J Evid Based Dent Pract. 2012;12(3):149-60.

2.   Botticelli D, Berglundh T, Lindhe J. Hard-tissue alterations following immediate implant placement in extraction sites. J Clin Periodontol. 2004;31(10):820-8.

3.   Schropp L, Wenzel A, Kostopoulos L, Karring T. Bone healing and soft tissue contour changes following single-tooth extraction: a clinical and radiographic 12-month prospective study.Int J Periodontics Restorative Dent. 2003;23(4):313-23.

4.   Tan WL, Wong TL, Wong MC, Lang NP. A systematic review of post-extractional alveolar hard and soft tissue dimensional changes in humans. Clin Oral Implants Res. 2012 Feb;23 Suppl 5:1-21.

5.   Prasad D, Shetty M, Bansal N, Hegde C. Crestal bone preservation: A review of different approaches for successful implant therapy. Indian J Dent Res. 2011;22(2):317-23.

6.   McKinney Jr RV, Steflik DE, Koth DL. The biologic response to the single-crystal sapphire endosteal dental implant: Scanning electron microscopic observations. J Prosthet Dent. 1984;51(3):372-9.

7.   Tadic D, Epple M. A thorough physicochemical characterisation of 14 calcium phosphate-based bone substitution materials in comparison to natural bone. Biomaterials. 2004;25(6):987-94.

8.   U. S. Department of Health and Human Services, Food and Drug Administration, Center for Drug Evaluation and Research, Center for Biologics Evaluation and Research. Q3D Elemental Impurities - Guidance for Industry [Internet]. 2015 [cited 2015 Nov 16]; Available from: http://www.fda.gov/downloads/drugs/guidancecomplianceregulatoryinformation/guidances/ ucm371025.pdf.

9.   European Commission. Commission Regulation (EC) No 1881/2006 of 19 December 2006 setting maximum levels for certain contaminants in foodstuffs. [Internet]. 2006 [cited 2016 Feb 15]; Available from: http://eur- lex.europa.eu/LexUriServ/LexUriServ.do?uri=OJ:L:2006:364:0005:0024:EN:PDF.

10.   European Commission. Commission Regulation (EU) No 420/2011 of 29 April 2011 amending Regulation (EC) No 1881/2006 setting maximum levels for certain contaminants in foodstuffs. [Internet]. 2011 [cited 2016 Feb 15]; Availablefrom   :   http://eur-lex.europa.eu/legal-content/PT/TXT/PDF/?uri=CELEX:32011R0420&from=EN.

11.   Dhandayuthapani B, Yoshida Y, Maekawa T, Kumar DS. Polymeric Scaffolds in Tissue Engineering Application: A Review. Int J Polym Sci. 2011.

12.   Barone A, Aldini NN, Fini M, Giardino R, Calvo Guirado JL, Covani U. Xenograft versus extraction alone for ridge preservation after tooth removal: a clinical and histomorphometric study. J Periodontol. 2008;79(8):1370-7.

13.   Camargo PM, Lekovic V, Weinlaender M, Klokkevold PR, Kenney EB, Dimitrijevic B, et al. Influence of bioactive glass on changes in alveolar process dimensions after exodontia. Oral Surg Oral Med Oral Pathol Oral Radiol Endod. 2000;90(5):581-6.

14.   Bolouri A, Haghighat N, Frederiksen N. Evaluation of the effect of immediate grafting of mandibular postextraction sockets with synthetic bone. Compend Contin Educ Dent. 2001;22(11):955-8.

15.   Pelegrine AA, Da Costa CES, Correa MEP, Marques JFC. Clinical and histomorphometric evaluation of extraction sockets treated with an autologous bone marrow graft. Clin Oral Implants Res. 2010;21(5):535-42.

16.   **Festa VM, Addabbo F, Laino L, Femiano F, Rullo R. Porcine-Derived Xenograft Combined** with a Soft Cortical Membrane versus Extraction Alone for Implant Site Development: A Clinical Study in Humans.Clin Implant Dent Relat Res. 2013;15(5):707-13.

17.   Cadman J, Zhou S, Chen Y, Li Q. Cuttlebone: Characterisation, Application and Development of Biomimetic Materials. J Bionic Eng. 2012;9(3):367-76.

18.   Rocha JHG, Lemos AF, Agathopoulos S, Valério P, Kannan S, Oktar FN, et al. Scaffolds for bone restoration from cuttlefish. Bone. 2005;37(6):850-7.

19.   Murugan R, Ramakrishna S, Panduranga Rao K. Nanoporous hydroxy-carbonate apatite scaffold made of natural bone. Mater Lett. 2006;60(23):2844-7.

20. Birchall JD, Thomas NL. On the architecture and function of cuttlefish bone. J Mater Sci. 1983;18(7):2081-6.

21. Gower D, Vincent JFV. The mechanical design of the cuttlebone and its bathymetric implications. Biomimetics. 1996;4:37-57.

22. Wiesmann HP, Joos U, Meyer U. Biological and biophysical principles in extracorporeal bone tissue engineering. Part II. Int J Oral Maxillofac Surg. 2004;33(6):523-30.

23. Rocha JHG, Lemos AF, Agathopoulos S, Kannan S, Valério P, Ferreira JMF. Hydrothermal growth of hydroxyapatite scaffolds from aragonitic cuttlefish bones. J Biomed Matr Res Part A. 2006;77A(1):160-8.

24. **Dogan E, Okumu§ Z. Cuttlebone used as a bone xenograft in bone healing.** Vet Med- Czech. 2014;59(5):254-60.

25. Ivankovic H, Gallego Ferrer G, Tkalcec E, Orlic S, Ivankovic M. Preparation of highly porous hydroxyapatite from cuttlefish bone. J Mater Sci Mater Med. 2009;20(5):1039-46.

26. **Okumu§ Z, Yildirim OS. The Cuttlefish Backbone: A New** Bone Xenograft Material? Turk J Vet Anim Sci. 2005;29(5):1177-84.

27. Mizuno M, Fukunaga K. Analysis of tissue condition based on interaction between inorganic and organic matter in cuttlefish bone. J Biol Phys. 2013;39(1):123-30.

28. Yildirim OS, Okumus Z, Kizilkaya M, Ozdemir Y, Durak R, Okur A. Comparative quantitative analysis of sodium, magnesium, potassium and calcium in healthy cuttlefish backbone and non- pathological human elbow bone. Can J Anal Sci Spect. 2007;52:270-5.

29. Jasso-Gastinel CF, Enriquez SG, Flores J, Reyes-González I, Mijares EM. Acrylic Bone Cements Modified With Bioactive Filler. Macromol Symp. 2009;283-284(1):159-66.

30. Garcia-Enriquez S, Guadarrama HE, Reyes-Gonzalez I, Mendizabal E, Jasso-Gastinel CF, Garcia-Enriquez B, et al. Mechanical performance and in vivo tests of an acrylic bone cement filled with bioactive sepia officinalis cuttlebone.J Biomater Sci Polym Ed. 2010;21:113-25.

31. Kannan S, Rocha JHG, Agathopoulos S, Ferreira JMF. Fluorine-substituted hydroxyapatite scaffolds hydrothermally grown from aragonitic cuttlefish bones. Acta Biomater. 2007;3(2):243-9.

32. Habraken W, Habibovic P, Epple M, Bohner M. Calcium phosphates in biomedical applications: materials for the future? Mater Today. 2016;19(2):69-87.

33. Milovac D, Gallego Ferrer G, Ivankovic M, Ivankovic H. PCL-coated hydroxyapatite scaffold derived from cuttlefish bone: morphology, mechanical properties and bioactivity. Mater Sci Eng C Mater Biol Appl. 2014;34:437-45.

34. Hongmin L, Wei Z, Xingrong Y, Jing W, Wenxin G, Jihong C, et al. Osteoinductive nanohydroxyapatite bone substitute prepared via in situ hydrothermal transformation of cuttlefish bone. J Biomed Matr Res Part B: Applied Biomaterials. 2015;103(4):816-24.

35. Calandrelli L, Immirzi B, Malinconico M, Orsello G, Volpe M, Ragione FD, et al. Biocompatibility studies on biodegradable polyester-based composites of human osteoblasts: A preliminary screening. J Biomed Matr Res. 2002;59(4):611-7.

36. Shamsuria O, Fadilah A, Asiah A, Rodiah M, Suzina A, Samsudin A. In vitro cytotoxicity evaluation

of biomaterials on human osteoblast cells CRL-1543; hydroxyapatite, natural coral and polyhydroxybutarate. Med J Malaysia. 2004;59:174-5.

37.   Jaishankar M, Tseten T, Anbalagan N, Mathew BB, Beeregowda KN. Toxicity, mechanism and health effects of some heavy metals. Interdiscip Toxicol. 2014;7(2):60-72.

38.   Cardellicchio N, Buccolieri A, di Leo A, Spada L. Heavy Metals in Marine Sediments from the Mar Piccolo of Taranto (Ionian Sea, Southern Italy). Ann Chim. 2006;96(11-12):727-41.

39.   Desideri D, Meli MA, Roselli C. A biomonitoring study: 210Po and heavy metals in marine organisms from the Adriatic Sea (Italy). J Radioanal Nucl Chem. 2010;285(2):373-82.

40.   Decleir W, Vlaeminck A, Geladi P, Van Grieken R. Determination of protein-bound copper and zinc in some organs of the cuttlefish Sepia officinalis L. Comp Biochem Physiol Part B Comparative Biochemistry. 1978;60(4):347-50.

41.   Miramand P, Bentley D. Concentration and distribution of heavy metals in tissues of two cephalopods, Eledone cirrhosa and Sepia officinalis, from the French coast of the English Channel. Mar Biol. 1992;114(3):407-14.

42.   Bustamante P. Etude des processus de bioaccumulation et de détoxication d'éléments traces (métaux lourds et terres rares) chez les mollusques céphalopodes et bivalves pectinidés. Implication of their bioavailability for transfer to predators. Implication of their bioavailability for transfer to predators. PhD [thesis]. University of La Rochelle France. 1998.

43.   Miramand P, Bustamante P, Bentley D, Kouéta N. Variation of heavy metal concentrations (Ag, Cd, Co, Cu, Fe, Pb, V, and Zn) during the life cycle of the common cuttlefish Sepia officinalis. Sci Total Environ. 2006;361(1):132-43.

44.   Kadouche S, Zemmouri H, Benaoumeur K, Drouiche N, Sharrock P, Lounici H. Metal Ion Binding on Hydroxyapatite (Hap) and Study of the Velocity of Sedimentation. Procedia Eng. 2012;33:377-84.

45.   del Rio JG, Sanchez P, Morando PJ, Cicerone DS. Retention of Cd, Zn and Co on hydroxyapatite filters. Chemosphere. 2006;64(6):1015-20.

46.   Suzuki T, Hatsushika T, Hayakawa Y. Synthetic hydroxyapatites employed as inorganic cation-exchangers. J Chem Soc Faraday Trans: Physical Chemistry in Condensed Phases. 1981;77(5):1059-62.

47.   Carroll SA, Bruno J. Mineral-solution interactions in the U (VI)-CO2-H2O system. Radiochim Acta. 1991;52(1):187-94.

48.   Reichert J, Binner J. An evaluation of hydroxyapatite-based filters for removal of heavy metal ions from aqueous solutions. J Mater Sci. 1996;31(5):1231-41.

49.   Chen X, Wright JV, Conca JL, Peurrung LM. Effects of pH on heavy metal sorption on mineral apatite. Environ Sci Technol. 1997;31(3):624-31.

50.   Vega E, Pedregosa J, Narda G. Interaction of oxovanadium (IV) with crystalline calcium hydroxyapatite: surface mechanism with no structural modification. J Phys Chem Solids. 1999;60(6):759-66.

51.   Leyva A, Marrero J, Smichowski P, Cicerone D. Antimony sorption on hydroxyapatite suspended in aqueous solutions. Environ Sci Technol. 2001;35:3669-75.

52.   McGrellis S, Serafini J-N, JeanJean J, Pastol J-L, Fedoroff M. Influence of the sorption protocol on

the uptake of cadmium ions in calcium hydroxyapatite. Separ Purif Technol. 2001;24(1):129-38.

53.	Wang Y, Chen T, Yeh K, Shue M. Stabilisation of an elevated heavy metal contaminated site. J Hazard Mater. 2001;88(1):63-74.

54.	Fuller C, Bargar J, Davis J, Piana M. Mechanisms of uranium interactions with hydroxyapatite: Implications for groundwater remediation. Environ Sci Technol. 2002;36(2):158- 65.

55.	Czerniczyniec M, Farias S, Magallanes J, Cicerone D, editors. Arsenic adsorption on biogenic PAH: solution composition effects. 11th International Conference on Surface and Colloid Science, Foz do Iguazu, Brazil; 2003.

56.	**del Rio JG, Morando P, Cicerone D. Natural materials for treatment of industrial** effluents: comparative study of the retention of Cd, Zn and Co by calcite and hydroxyapatite. Part I: batch experiments. J Environ Manage. 2004;71(2):169-77.

57.	Zhang Z, Li M, Chen W, Zhu S, Liu N, Zhu L. Immobilisation of lead and cadmium from aqueous solution and contaminated sediment using nano-hydroxyapatite. Environ Pollut. 2010;158(2):514-9.

58.	Mobasherpour I, Salahi E, Pazouki M. Removal of divalent cadmium cations by means of synthetic nano crystallite hydroxyapatite. Desalination Water Treat. 2011;266(1):142-8.

59.	He M, Shi H, Zhao X, Yu Y, Qu B. Immobilisation of Pb and Cd in contaminated soil using nano-crystallite hydroxyapatite. Procedia Environ Sci. 2013;18:657-65.

60.	Taneez M, Marmier N, Hurel C. Use of neutralised industrial residue to stabilize trace elements (Cu, Cd, Zn, As, Mo, and Cr) in marine dredged sediment from South-East of France. Chemosphere. 2016;150:116-22.

61.	Mignardi S, Corami A, Ferrini V. Evaluation of the effectiveness of phosphate treatment for the remediation of mine waste soils contaminated with Cd, Cu, Pb, and Zn. Chemosphere. 2012;86(4):354-60.

62.	Shen Q, Luo L, Bian L, Liu Y, Yuan B, Liu C, et al. Lead cations immobilisation by hydroxyapatite with cotton-like morphology. J Alloys Compd. 2016;673:175-81.

63.	**Smiciklas I, Onjia A, Raicevic S, Janackovic D, Mitric M. Factors influencing the removal of** divalent cations by hydroxyapatite. J Hazard Mater. 2008;152(2):876-84.

64.	Kaludjerovic-Radoicic T, Raicevic S. Aqueous Pb sorption by synthetic and natural apatite: kinetics, equilibrium and thermodynamic studies. Chem Eng J. 2010;160(2):503-10.

65.	Zhu R, Yu R, Yao J, Mao D, Xing C, Wang D. Removal of Cd 2+ from aqueous solutions by hydroxyapatite. Catal Today. 2008;139(1):94-9.

66.	Corami A, Mignardi S, Ferrini V. Cadmium removal from single-and multi-metal (Cd+ Pb+ Zn+ Cu) solutions by sorption on hydroxyapatite. J Colloid Interface Sci. 2008;317(2):402-8.

67.	Sheha R. Sorption behaviour of Zn (II) ions on synthesized hydroxyapatites. J Colloid Interface Sci. 2007;310(1):18-26.

68.	Corami A, Mignardi S, Ferrini V. Copper and zinc decontamination from single-and binary-metal solutions using hydroxyapatite. J Hazard Mater. 2007;146(1):164-70.

69.	**Sljivic M, Smiciklas I, Plecas I, Mitric M. The influence of equilibration conditions and** hydroxyapatite physico-chemical properties onto retention of Cu 2+ ions. Chem Eng J. 2009;148(1):80-8.

70.   **Smiciklas I, Dimovic S, Plecas I, Mitric M. Removal of Co 2+ from aqueous Solutions by** hydroxyapatite. Water Res. 2006;40(12):2267-74.

71.   **Corami A, D'Acapito F, Mignardi S, Ferrini V. Removal of Cu from aqueous Solutions by** synthetic hydroxyapatite: EXAFS investigation. Mater Sci Eng C Mater Bio Appl. 2008;149(2):209- 13.

72.   Linhart W, Briem D, Amling M, Rueger JM, Windolf J. Mechanisches Versagen einer porosen Hydroxylapatitkeramik 7,5 Jahre nach Implantation an der proximalen Tibia. Der Unfallchirurg.107(2):154-7.

73.   Doi Y, Shibutani T, Moriwaki Y, Kajimoto T, Iwayama Y. Sintered carbonate apatites as bioresorbable bone substitutes. J Biomed Mater Res. 1998;39(4):603-10.

74.   Dersot JM, Colombier ML, Lafont J, Baroukh B, Septier D, Saffar JL. Multinucleated giant cells elicited around hydroxyapatite particles implanted in craniotomy defects are not osteoclasts. Anat Rec. 1995;242(2):166-76.

75.   Ayukawa Y, Suzuki Y, Tsuru K, Koyano K, Ishikawa K. Histological Comparison in Rats between Carbonate Apatite Fabricated from Gypsum and Sintered Hydroxyapatite on Bone Remodelling. BioMed Res Int. 2015;2015:7.

76.   Moore WR, Graves SE, Bain GI. Synthetic bone graft substitutes. ANZ J Surg. 2001;71(6):354-61.

77.   Legeros RZ. Biodegradation and bioresorption of calcium phosphate ceramics. Clin Mater. 1993;14(1):65-88.

78.   Fulmer MT, Ison IC, Hankermayer CR, Constantz BR, Ross J. Measurements of the solubilities and dissolution rates of several hydroxyapatites. Biomaterials. 2002;23(3):751-5.

79.   Gu Y-G, Lin Q, Yu Z-L, Wang X-N, Ke C-L, Ning J-J. Speciation and risk of heavy metals in sediments and human health implications of heavy metals in edible nekton in Beibu Gulf, China: A case study of Qinzhou Bay. Marine Poll Bull. 2015;101(2):852-9.

80.   Gao X, Chen C-TA. Heavy metal pollution status in surface sediments of the coastal Bohai Bay. Water Res. 2012;46(6):1901-11.

81.   Gleyzes C, Tellier S, Astruc M. Fractionation studies of trace elements in contaminated soils and sediments: a review of sequential extraction procedures. Trac-Trends Anal Chem. 2002;21(6):451-67.

82.   Sutherland RA. BCR®-701: A review of 10-years of sequential extraction analyses. Anal Chim Acta. 2010;680(1):10-20.

83.   Le Bihan E, Perrin A, Koueta N. Development of a bioassay from isolated digestive gland cells of the cuttlefish Sepia officinalis L.(Mollusca Cephalopoda): effect of Cu, Zn and Ag on enzyme activities and cell viability. J Exp Mar Bio Eco. 2004;309(1):47-66.

84.   Seixas FLS. Analysis of Heavy Metals in Redfish (Chelidonichthys lucernus, LINNAEUS, 1758). Porto: University of Porto; 2008.

85.   Salbu B, Steinnes E. Trace Elements in the oceans. In: J. R. Donat, Bruland KW, editors. Trace Elements in Natural Waters. Boca Raton, Florida: CRC-Press; 1995. p. 247-81.

86.   Millero FJ. Chemical Oceanography. 3§ ed. Miami: CRC Press; 2006.

87.   World Health Organisation. Cadmium - Environmental Health Criteria 134 [Internet]. 2015[cited2016Feb29   ];Av   ail   able from: http://www.inchem.org/documents/ehc/ehc/ehc134.htm.

88.   Agency for Toxic Substances and Disease Registry. Toxicological profile for Cadmium. US Department of Health and Human Services, Public Health Service. [Internet] Atlanta. 1999 [cited 2016 29 Feb]; Available from: http://www.atsdr.cdc.gov/toxprofiles/tp5.pdf.

89.   World Health Organisation. Copper. Environmental Health Criteria 200. [Internet]. 2015 [cited 2016 Mar 6]; Available from: http://www.inchem.org/documents/ehc/ehc/ehc200.htm.

90.   Roychoudhury S, Nath S, Massanyi P, Stawarz R, Kacaniova M, Kolesarova A. Copper induced changes in reproductive functions: review of in vivo and in vitro effects. Physiol Res. 2015; 65(1).

91.   Sprague JB. Toxicity and tissue concentrations of lead, zinc, and cadmium for marine molluscs and crustaceans. Research Triangle Park, NC: International Lead Zinc Research Organisation. 1987.

92.   World Health Organisation. Zinc. Environment Health Criteria 221. [Internet]. 2015 [cited 2016 Mar 9]; Available from: http://www.inchem.org/documents/ehc/ehc/ehc221.htm.

93.   United States Environment Protection Agency. Ambient water quality criteria for zinc - 1987. United States Environment Protection Agency Report 440/5-87-003. 1987:1-207.

94.   Yeats PA. The distribution of trace metals in ocean waters. Sci Total Environ. 1988;72:131-49.

CHAPTER 7

Annexes

Metal	Ocean concentration	Maximum quantity allowed in cephalopods according to Regulation (EC) No 1881/2006 (9), as amended in 2011 by Regulation (EU) No 420/2011 (10)
Lead	Average levels are around 0.005 μg/L. (84) In the Atlantic Ocean, it ranges from 100 pmol/kg to 150 pmol/kg in surface waters and 20 pmol/kg in deeper waters (84-86).	1.0 μg/g fresh weight for cephalopods intended for human consumption, without viscera.
Cadmium	It can range from 0.01 to O.lmg/L (84, 87, 88); In the North Atlantic Ocean, it varies between 100 and 200 pmol/kg at the surface and in deeper waters it reaches 300 pmol/kg (85, 86).	1.0 μg/g fresh weight for cephalopods intended for human consumption, without viscera.
Mercury	It varies between 1 and 7 pmol/kg in the most superficial zones and in deep waters it is approximately 1 pmol/kg. (85)	0.50 μg/g fresh weight for cephalopods intended for human consumption, without viscera.
Copper	Approximately 0.15 μg/L. (89)	N.D. According to the WHO, the maximum daily intake of copper may be more than 2-3 mg. (90)
Zinc	It varies between 0.0005-0.026 μg/L (91, 92), with values between 0.002-0.1 μg/L in open waters. (93) In the North Atlantic Ocean, the concentration at 20 metres depth is 0.065μpg/L and at 3715 metres it is 0.124μg/L. (92, 94)	N.D. The amount of zinc incorporated into the human body, taking into account all the sources through which this intake can occur, will be approximately 4.7 to 16 mg per day, with food being the main source. (92)

Annex II - Statistical treatment of Pb spectrometry readings

Group	Concentration (μg/g)	Average (μg/g)	Standard deviation (μg/g)
A1	32	331667	4,87511
	33		
	30		
	27		
	41		
	36		
	20		

Group		Average	Standard deviation
A2	20 18 18 18 15	18,1667	1,83485
BI	30 29 26 29 26 27	27,8333	1,72240
B2	18 20 22 14 20 13	17,8333	3,60093

Descriptive Statistics

	N	Minimum	Maximum	Average	Standard Deviation
LeadAl	6	27,00	41,00	33,1667	4,87511
LeadA2	6	15,00	20,00	18,1667	1,83485
LeadBl	6	26,00	30,00	27,8333	1,72240
LeadB2	6	13,00	22,00	17,8333	3,60093
N valid (listwise)	6				

Annex III - Statistical treatment of Cu spectrometry readings

Group	Concentration (µg/g)	Average (µg/g)	Standard deviation (µg/g)
A1	4,8 4,9 5,1 4,8 4,6 4,8	48333	0,16330
A2	5,5 5,5 5,2 5,0 5,0 4,9	5,1833	0,26394
BI	4,0 4,1 4,0 3,9 4,1 3,9	4,0000	0,08944
B2	4,2 4,2 4,2	4,1667	0,08165

| 4,2 |
| 4,2 |
| 4,0 |

Descriptive Statistics

	N	Minimum	Maximum	Average	Standard Deviation
CopperAl	6	4,60	5,10	4,8333	,16330
Copper A2	6	4,90	5,50	5,1833	,26394
CobreBl	6	3,90	4,10	4,0000	,08944
CopperB2	6	4,00	4,20	4,1667	,08165
N valid (listwise)	6				

Annex IV - Statistical treatment of Cd spectrometry readings

Group	Concentration (µg/g)	Average (µg/g)	Standard deviation (µg/g)
A1	<0,4 <0,4 <0,4 <0,4 <0,4 <0,4	<0,4	N.D
A2	1,7 1,1 1,1 1,3 1,3 1,8	1,3833	0,29944
BI	<0,3 <0,3 <0,3 <0,3 <0,3 <0,3	<0,3	N.D
B2	0,9 0,7 0,8 0,5 0,5 1,1	0,7500	0,23452

Descriptive Statistics

	N	Minimum	Maximum	Average	Standard Deviation
CadmiumAl	0				
CadmiumA2	6	1,10	1,80	1,3833	,29944
CadmiumBl	0				
CadmiumB2	6	,50	1,10	,7500	,23452
N valid (listwise)	0				

Annex V - Statistical treatment of Zn spectrometry readings

Group	Concentration	Average	Standard deviation

	(µg/g)	(µg/g)	(µg/g)
AI	19 20 19	19,3333	0,57735
A2	22 23 23	22,6667	0,57735
BI	34 33 34	33,6667	0,57735
B2	44 42 44	43,3333	1,15470

Descriptive Statistics

	N	Minimum	Maximum	Average	Standard Deviation
ZincAl	3	19,00	20,00	19,3333	,57735
ZincA2	3	22,00	23,00	22,6667	,57735
ZincBl	3	33,00	34,00	33,6667	,57735
ZincB2	3	42,00	44,00	43,3333	1,15470
N valid (listwise)	3				

Annex VI - Statistical treatment of Hg spectrometry readings

Group	Concentration (µg/g)	Average (µg/g)	Standard deviation (µg/g)
AI	< 28 < 28 < 28	< 28	N.D.
A2	< 34 < 34 < 34	< 34	N.D.
BI	< 22 < 22 < 22	< 22	N.D.
B2	< 34 < 34 < 34	< 34	N.D

Annex VII - Statistical treatment of the comparison of concentrations between groups of samples without (A1) and with hydrothermal processing (A2), taken at the same location A

Mann-Whitney test

Posts

	Group	N	Medium post	Sum of Posts
Concentration_Pb	A1	6	9,50	57,00
	A2	6	3,50	21,00
	Total	12		

Concentration_Cu	A1	6	4,08	24,50
	A2	6	8,92	53,50
	Total	12		
Zn_concentration	A1	3	2,00	6,00
	A2	3	5,00	15,00
	Total	6		

Test statisticsa

	Concentration_ Pb	Concentration_ Cu	Concentration_ Zn
Mann-Whitney U	,000	3,500	,000
Wilcoxon W	21,000	24,500	6,000
Z	-2,908	-2,351	-2,023
Significance Assint. (Bilateral)	**,004**	**,019**	**,043**
Exact Sig [2*(One-sided Sig)]	,002[b]	,015[b]	, 100[b]

a. Grouping Variable: Group b. Not corrected for ties.

Annex VIII - Statistical treatment of the comparison of concentrations between groups of samples without (B1) and with hydrothermal processing (B2), taken at the same location B

Mann-Whitney test

Posts

	Group	N	Medium post	Sum of Posts
Concentration_Pb	B1	6	9,50	57,00
	B2	6	3,50	21,00
	Total	12		
Concentration_Cu	B1	6	4,00	24,00
	B2	6	9,00	54,00
	Total	12		
Zn_concentration	B1	3	2,00	6,00
	B2	3	5,00	15,00
	Total	6		

Test statisticsa

	Concentration_ Pb	Concentration_ Cu	Concentration_ Zn
Mann-Whitney U	,000	3,000	,000
Wilcoxon W	21,000	24,000	6,000
Z	-2,898	-2,519	-2,023
Significance Assint. (Bilateral)	**,004**	**,012**	**,043**
Exact Sig [2*(Sig. of one-sided)]	,002[b]	,015[b]	, 100[b]

a. Grouping Variable: Group b. Not corrected for ties.

Annex IX - Statistical treatment of the comparison of concentrations between groups of samples without hydrothermal processing (A1 and B1), taken at different locations A and B

Mann-Whitney test

Posts

	Group	N	Medium post	Sum of Posts
Concentration_Pb	A1	6	8,83	53,00
	B1	6	4,17	25,00

		N	Medium post	Sum of Posts
	Total	12		
Concentration_Cu	A1	6	9,50	57,00
	B1	6	3,50	21,00
	Total	12		
Zn_concentration	A1	3	2,00	6,00
	B1	3	5,00	15,00
	Total	6		

Test statisticsa

	Concentration_ Pb	Concentration_ Cu	Concentration_ Zn
Mann-Whitney U	4,000	,000	,000
Wilcoxon W	25,000	21,000	6,000
Z	-2,258	-2,918	-2,023
Significance Assint. (Bilateral)	**,024**	**,004**	**,043**
Exact Sig [2*(One-sided Sig)]	,026[b]	,002[b]	, 100[b]

a. Grouping Variable: Group b. Not corrected for ties.

Annex X - Statistical treatment of the comparison of concentrations between groups of samples with hydrothermal processing (A2 and B2), taken at different locations A and B

Mann-Whitney test

Posts

	Group	N	Medium post	Sum of Posts
Concentration_Pb	A2	6	6,42	38,50
	B2	6	6,58	39,50
	Total	12		
Concentration_Cu	A2	6	9,50	57,00
	B2	6	3,50	21,00
	Total	12		
Zn_concentration	A2	3	2,00	6,00
	B2	3	5,00	15,00
	Total	6		
Concentration_Cd	A2	6	9,33	56,00
	B2	6	3,67	22,00
	Total	12		

Test statisticsa

	Concentration_ Pb	Concentration_ Cu	Concentration_ Zn	Concentration_ Cd
Mann-Whitney U	17,500	,000	,000	1,000
Wilcoxon W	38,500	21,000	6,000	22,000
Z	-,083	-3,000	-2,023	-2,751
Significance Assint. (Bilateral)	**,934**	**,003**	**,043**	**,006**
Exact Sig [2*(One-sided Sig)]	,037[h]	,002[h]	, 100[h]	,004[h]

a. Grouping Variable: Group b. Not corrected for ties.

Annex XI - Limit concentrations established by the FDA (8)

Metal	Permissible daily exposure via parenteral route (µg/day)	Permissible concentrations for impurities in pharmaceutical products, substances and excipients, valid for parenteral administration not exceeding 10 g per day

		(µg/day)
Lead	5	0,5
Cadmium	2	0,2
Mercury	3	0,3
Copper	300	30
Zinc	It doesn't exist	It doesn't exist

The FDA provides for situations in which there are higher concentrations of metals in drugs and derivatives, particularly in cases of single administration, such as the implantation of HA obtained from cuttlefish bone in alveoli immediately after tooth extraction.

Annex XII - Declaration of authorisation from the Directorate-General for Food and Veterinary Products

Dear Sir(s),

In response to your e-mail of 25.02.2016, regarding the request for authorisation for the collection, transport and use of category 3 animal by-products from local fishmongers in the city of Aveiro, namely cuttlefish bone/shell for specific research purposes, we inform you that under the provisions of Article 17 of Regulation (EC) No 1069/2009, the handling and use of category 3 animal by-products for research purposes is authorised.§, that under the provisions of Article 17 of Regulation (EC) No 1069/2009 of 21 October, the handling and use of category 3 animal by-products for research purposes is authorised, provided that the following conditions are met to ensure the control of risks to public and animal health:

> The operator of animal by-products for diagnosis and research must take all necessary measures to prevent the spread of diseases transmissible to humans or animals during the handling of the material under his responsibility, in particular by applying good laboratory practices.
> Any subsequent use of animal by-products for purposes other than examination in the context of authorised activities is prohibited.
> Transport to the final destination must be carried out in packaging, vehicles or containers suitable for the purpose and labelled "Category 3 - For research and diagnosis";
> Unless they are kept for reference purposes, diagnostic and research samples, and any products derived from the use of these samples, must be disposed of:

   a) As waste, by incineration or coincineration;

   b) In the case of animal by-products or derived products referred to in Article 8(a)(iv), Article 8(c) and (d), Article 9 and Article 10 of Regulation (EC) No 1069/2009 which are part of cell cultures, laboratory kits or laboratory samples, by treatment under conditions which are at least equivalent to the validated method for steam autoclaves [1] and subsequent disposal as waste or waste water in accordance with the relevant Union legislation.

   [1] CEN TC/102 - Sterilisers for medical purposes - EN 285:2006 + A2:2009 - Sterilisation - Steam sterilisers - Large sterilisers; reference published in OJ C 293, 2.12.2009, p. 39.

   c) By pressure sterilisation and subsequent disposal or use in accordance with Articles 12, 13 and 14 of Regulation (EC) No 1069/2009.

   d) The user must keep a dated record of the animal by-products used, which must specify the description of the material, animal species, category, quantity, date, place of origin, name of the consignor, name of the user and method of disposal of the samples and any derived products.

Notice is hereby given that, under the terms of Article 23(1)(a) of Regulation (EC) No 1069/2009 of 21 October, the **FACULDADE DE MEDICINA DENTÁRIA DA UNIVERSIDADE DO PORTO**, located at Rua Dr. Manuel Pereira da Silva, 4200-393 Porto, has been assigned registration number **N.15.061.UDER,** as a user of category 3 animal by-products for research purposes.

Best regards,

José M. Correia
Agr. Techn. Eng.
DGAV - General Directorate of Food and Veterinary Science
DCCA - Food Chain Control Division
Quinta do Marquês, AvJ República, 2780-155 Oeiras
Tef. General: 21 446 40 00 Tef. Secret. 21 446 40 61
Fax: 21 446 40 99 e-mail: jmcorreia@dgav.pt

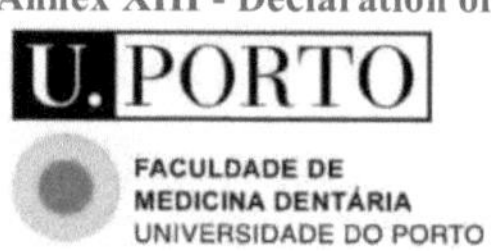

**FACULDADE DE
MEDICINA DENTÁRIA**
UNIVERSIDADE DO PORTO

DECLARATION
Research Monograph

I declare that this work, within the scope of the Research Monograph, integrated in the MIMD, of the FMDUP, is my own and that all sources have been duly referenced.

25/05/2016

The Investigator

Carlos Miguel Silva Sousa Veiga

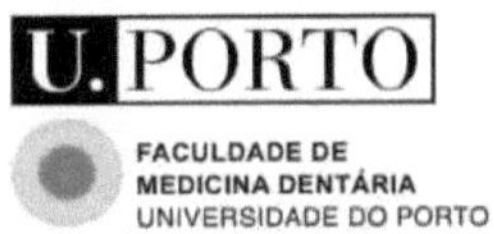

**FACULDADE DE
MEDICINA DENTÁRIA
UNIVERSIDADE DO PORTO**

OPINION

In my capacity as supervisor of the Integrated Master's thesis **developed by Carlos Miguel Silva Sousa Veiga, entitled "Cuttlefish Bone as a Biomaterial in Dental Medicine", I would like to** inform you that I have checked it and give my opinion:

- The research work is timely, well-structured, methodologically appropriate and well-developed.

- The dissertation complies with all scientific and written presentation standards, presents the topic clearly, correctly defines the objectives it sets out to achieve, presents a very complete introduction and the materials and methods are thoroughly described. The bibliography is related to the research topic.

- The candidate is scheduled to submit an international publication.

- Thus, the candidate is able to present the monograph and take public exams.

Porto, 23rd May 2016

The supervisor,

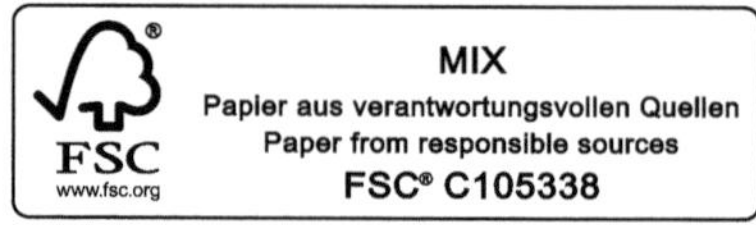

Printed by Books on Demand GmbH, Norderstedt / Germany